Sandbag Training

Build a Fit & Functional Body Using Workouts That Are Efficient and Effective

Thomas Rohmer

Copyright © 2018

Disclaimer:

This guide has been created for informational and reference purposes only. The author, publisher, and any other affiliated parties cannot be held in any way accountable for any personal injuries or damage allegedly resulting from the information contained herein, or from any misuse of such guidance. Although strict measures have been taken to provide accurate information, the parties involved with the creation and publication of this guide take no responsibility for any issues that many arise from alleged discrepancies contained herein. It is strongly recommended that you consult a physician, personal trainer, and nutritionist prior to commencing this or any other workout or diet plan. This guide is not a substitute for professional personal guidance from a qualified medical professional. If you feel pain or discomfort at any point during exercises contained herein, cease the activity immediately and seek medical guidance.

Before You Begin:

Bonus Gift: Free Exercise Demonstration Video

As a thanks for picking up this book, I'd love to give you a free gift exclusive to my readers that'll help you get results even faster!

I created a free video where I personally demonstrate how to perform each and every exercise that's in this book.

With this video guide, you'll be able to ensure that you're doing all of the exercises correctly, which will help you maximize your results with this book.

Visit the link below to instantly download the video demonstration guide:

https://rohmerfitness.lpages.co/sandbag-exercise-guide/

Table of Contents

Introduction:

Sandbag training is awesome! Seriously not enough people take advantage of the many benefits that sandbag training can provide you with.

It's not an expensive or sexy piece of equipment (it's a bag with sand in it for crying out loud!), but trust me sandbag workouts are some of the most intense workouts you'll ever do. And once you have a sandbag, you can do a wide variety of exercises that will work all of the different muscle groups in your body.

Sandbag training really is a no-brainer! Sadly sandbag training doesn't cross the minds of many people that workout. They might falsely think that you can't hit your muscles as good with a sandbag than you can with a dumbbell or barbell.

As you're about to find out, you can actually get a more effective workout with a simple sandbag than you can with a regular barbell or dumbbell. Don't be fooled into thinking that just because a certain piece of fitness equipment is more popular (such as a barbell) that automatically means that it's better. Be smart and train efficiently and effectively with one of the best-kept secrets in the fitness industry—the sandbag!

Section 1: 7 Reasons Why Sandbag Training is Awesome

Reason 1: Your Body is Always Guessing

My favorite thing about training with a sandbag is the fact that the weight of the bag shifts. When you first start to train with a sandbag, you'll feel awkward in how you handle the bag.

If all you're used to is training with dumbbells and barbells, then you'll definitely feel out of place when you train with a sandbag. This is because you'll fill a bag with sand, and then that sand will be shifting around the bag when you workout with it.

You might be thinking, "Ok that's cool and all, but why does that matter?" Well, think about it. Whenever you do a bicep curl with a dumbbell for example, the distribution of the weight is always the same.

Therefore your body will adapt and know exactly what you're up to. You must constantly adapt your workouts to keep your body guessing so that you'll continue to get results. The body will only adapt to stresses and demands that it has to. If it knows what's coming, then there's no need to adapt, which means no more results for you.

This is how your body works in regards to building new muscle, getting in better shape, etc. When you go to the gym, you workout and break down your muscle. The workout that you did was a stimulus or stress for your body.

Your body just wants to maintain the status quo. It wants to stay the same; your body doesn't want to make changes.

However, you just did a workout in the gym, so your body is going to be like, "Wow that was intense, I never want to experience that again!" Your body is then going to build new muscle to help prepare it for the future when it might face that stimulus again.

It's during the recovery phase (i.e. when you are resting and not working out) that your body actually rebuilds itself back up bigger and stronger. Therefore, your body adapts to stresses that you place it under.

So what happens if you keep placing your body under the same stresses? As you can probably guess your body won't know what's going on at first, and this is where you'll notice some initial results. Then after a while, your body will adapt and know exactly what you're about to throw at it. At this point, your results will come to a stifling halt.

And this is where sandbag training comes into play. Let's say you're doing an exercise like a bicep curl with a sandbag instead of a dumbbell. What's the difference?

Well, the weight distribution in the sandbag will be different each and every time you curl the bag. The same can't be said for a dumbbell.

This means that your body will always be guessing and constantly having the adapt to the new stimulus. So yes sandbag training feels awkward and that's because it's supposed to!

Feeling uncomfortable or awkward is the best way to ensure that your body will never know what's going to happen next. The key to making sure this happens is to make sure that you don't overfill your sandbag.

You can buy a sandbag online or make your own, but either way, you don't want to overfill your sandbag. If you overfill your sandbag, then you won't give the sand in the bag enough room to be able to move around.

Instead, you'll basically be working out with the equivalent of a heavy brick! This isn't what we want because now the distribution of the weight will be the same every time and the body will be able to easily adapt.

That's why in my opinion it's easier to buy a sandbag online. This way you won't have to worry about the durability of the bag, and you also won't have to worry about the sand not having enough room to move.

I've seen people make sandbags buy going to the store and buying a bag of sand and then covering it with many layers of duct tape. This is a big mistake!

You're now working out with an oversized brick instead of a sandbag that allows for the sand to move, which is the entire point of sandbag training. Additionally, when you buy a sandbag, it'll come with handles on the sandbag.

This is a really nice feature that shouldn't be glossed over. If you make your own sandbag without handles, then you're going to be limited on what exercises you can and can't do.

Having handles across different positions on the bag will allow you to train and perform a series of different exercises with ease. And buying a sandbag really isn't that big of an investment, so it really is easier just to buy one online so you know it's ready to go and you can focus on what really matters which is the workouts.

Of course, if you want to make your own sandbag you certainly can, but just consider how much time you'll have to spend making it, and if you can make it sturdy enough but still serve the purpose of allowing the sand the shift in the bag.

Reason #2: Great for Functional Strength and Conditioning

I used to laugh when people would say that their training was "functional." I thought you just trained and that was that! But boy was I wrong!

What exactly does functional training mean anyway? It means exercising in a way that's practical and beneficial for whatever it is you're trying to do in life. What's functional for one person might be different for another person.

For example, what's functional training for a basketball player? Well believe it or not a typical game of basketball usually works out to where the players are engaging in intense activity for roughly 45 seconds and then they get to rest for 15 seconds.

So you might be playing really hard for 45 seconds, then the whistle blows when the ball goes out of bounds. The players will get to rest for 15 seconds or so while everyone gets reset and the team throws the ball back in play.

Therefore, functional training for a basketball player would be doing conditioning work where the player is working for 45 seconds and then taking a 15-second rest before starting the next round. That's just one example, but what if you're a regular person who's simply looking to get more fit—what's functional to you?

Well, think about things you regularly do: load and unload groceries, help a friend move furniture, carrying laundry baskets, moving bags of potting soil, etc. These are a few examples of things you'll do regularly throughout your life.

You'll be carrying bulky objects, objects that are weighted unevenly, etc. Therefore you still need to be prepared for the general activities of day-to-day life.

You might be thinking, "Well can't I get stronger by lifting weights using dumbbells and barbells?" The answer to that is yes you can, but remember what I talked about in the previous benefit of sandbag training.

When you use dumbbells for example, the weight distribution will always be the same. When you help a friend move furniture, is it always the same? No, it's never the same! Each piece of furniture will weigh a different amount and it will be shaped differently as well.

You'll need to know how to be able to adapt your body to be able to lift each and every different piece of furniture. You simply won't be able to do that if you lift using dumbbells or barbells all of the time.

This is where sandbag training comes into play. It's as close as it gets to mimicking daily tasks that you'll be doing in your life.

The sandbag's weight distribution is always different and thus it forces you to adapt to it each and every time. Of course, your body never knows what in the world is going on, just like how your body doesn't know what's going on when you're moving different sized bulky objects.

And this really is true. Most of my fitness career, I've lifted using dumbbells and barbells. When I'd have to help someone move though, I'd notice that I really struggled even though I would consider myself a pretty fit person.

Then when I started training using sandbags, I would totally get wiped out! It was something that my body wasn't used to at all!

I'd be completely spent in less than 10 minutes when I first started to incorporate sandbag training into my routine. I started to realize why I always got gassed when I would help my friends move or do something similar—my body wasn't used to that stimulus at all.

All it ever knew was dumbbells and barbells. My body was used to doing the same routine over and over again.

If I had to do a lifting competition with my friends in the bench press for example, I'd feel pretty confident. But if I had to go against a farmer lifting hay bells, I know I'd get crushed.

Think about it—why are farmers some of the strongest people in the world? It's because all they do is lift, carry, and move awkward and heavy objects all day! That's far more difficult than simply lifting some dumbbells for 30 minutes 3 times a week.

And the great thing is that sandbag training is similar to how a farmer lifts when he works! You want to actually be strong and fit, instead of just looking strong like how I was back in the day.

Reason #3: Workouts Can be Done Pretty Much Anywhere

What's one of the main problems with working out in a commercial gym? You have to change clothes and drive to the gym.

Depending on how far away you live from the gym, this can be a huge inconvenience. Then once you're at the gym, you have to worry about how crowded the gym is. If you go when it's packed, then there's a good chance that you'll have to wait to use the equipment.

This happened to me quite a bit when I worked out at a popular commercial gym. Think about it—if you work a regular job with regular hours, the best time to go to the gym for you is probably the same time as everyone else!

This makes it hard to be able to go to the gym and not have to worry about someone else hogging the equipment. Not only that but when you do finish your workout you still have to drive back home!

So all in all your 1-hour workout will take you a lot longer than 1 hour to complete. Compare that to working out with a sandbag.

The sandbag is one simple piece of equipment. It's not very big or bulky, so it can easily be taken with you wherever you go.

Thus, it's extremely simple to be able to workout wherever you want whenever you want. You could workout in your backyard or the comfort of your own home if you have space for it.

The point is convenience. The harder it is for you to start a workout, the less likely you are to do it.

And thinking about driving to a packed gym, having to wait to do certain exercises, and then having to drive back sounds like a pretty big pain in the neck! I know from experience firsthand how critical it is to make starting a workout as easy as possible.

One semester during college, I set up my schedule to where I didn't have any classes on Friday. I was super excited to always have a 3-day weekend!

However, my workout routine took a big hit that semester. Usually, I would take the bus from my apartment to campus, and then I would hit the gym after all of my classes were over with.

This worked out great because I already had a reason to be on campus due to my classes, and thus it was simple for me to walk to the rec center and workout. However, things became much different during that semester when I didn't schedule any Friday classes.

It was such a pain for me to have to workout that I ended up skipping my Friday workouts a lot of the times! I would have to walk to the bus stop (after sleeping in of course), wait for the bus, and then walk all way across campus to get to the rec center.

After my workout, I would have to walk all the way back across campus, wait on the bus, and then walk back to my apartment. Talk about annoying!

Thinking about having to do all of that to do a workout wasn't worth it to me a lot of the times so I would skip. Then the following semester, I decided to make a small tweak.

I decided to schedule one class on Friday. And I also made sure that the class was close by to the rec center.

This way when Friday rolled around, I had a reason to go to campus, and it was easy for me to get to the rec after class was over. Boom it was that simple!

I was able to workout all while maintaining a Friday class schedule that wasn't too hectic (no one wants that!). It's not that I was lazy one semester and highly motivated the following semester.

I changed things to make it more convenient. And since you're human like me, I'm sure you can relate to my situation. If you haven't consistently exercised throughout your life, I seriously doubt it's because you're lazy.

It probably has something to do with your P.E. teacher making you hate exercise. Or maybe you're sick and tired of boring workouts and no one taught you how to make exercise fun. Or maybe you're like me when I was in college and working out has always been super inconvenient for you.

Whatever your reason is or whatever your past, it doesn't matter. What matters is that sandbag training will make easy to workout (the workouts themselves will not be easy!), and it'll make working out fun again.

Seriously if working out feels like a grind, then any rational person is bound to quit sooner or later. Working out should be enjoyable and you should feel great after doing it!

So once you have a sandbag, you really don't have much of an excuse to not workout. As long as you have enough space for your body to be able to move in multiple planes and directions you should be good to go in most cases.

Of course, depending on what exercises you're doing, you might need more space sometimes. Generally, though, you won't need that much space in order to workout with a sandbag. That sure beats having to use a spare bedroom to fill with fitness equipment!

Reason #4: Better Than Bodyweight Training

Look bodyweight training is great no doubt about it, but the thing is that there are some major cons to it. Yes, it's great that bodyweight training can be done anytime anywhere, however the biggest flaw with bodyweight training is progression.

Additionally, you're also very limited in exercise selection, which means that you're probably going to get bored after a while. This is critical because of a principle called progressive overload.

Essentially this means that you must always be doing more in order for your body to keep growing bigger and stronger. Let's use the bench press as an example. If you start a new workout routine and can bench press 135 pounds, and then 3 months later you're still bench pressing 135 pounds, you're not going to be getting any results.

Instead, you must progressively overload your body overtime by either increasing the weight, increasing the number of reps that you can do, or by decreasing rest time. So for example, if in March you can bench press 135 pounds, and then in April you increase your bench press to 150 pounds, this means that you're on the right track and are getting stronger and should be getting bigger as well.

And that's the big problem with bodyweight training. Yes, it's possible to progressively overload your body with bodyweight exercises, but it's really hard to do so. Think about it—if you want to progressively overload your body with the bench press you can do so in steady increments of 5 pounds.

However, with a push-up how do you overload that exercise? You can certainly do more reps, but at a certain point that gets to be a little repetitive and diminishing. Imagining having to do 50+ pushups every set just to get a good workout in!

You'd essentially have to do an insane amount of reps for the workout to even be worthwhile. The other thing you could do is go from a two-arm pushup to a one-arm pushup.

But this is a pretty hard progression to make. There are a lot of people out there who can easily knock out 50 two-arm pushups in a row, but they can't do a single one-arm push-up. The same can be said for bodyweight squats.

You could get to the point to where you could do 50 bodyweight squats in a row, but then when it's time to take things up a notch are you going to be able to do a single-legged squat? Maybe you can maybe you can't. The point is that with bodyweight training the jumps in how you overload the exercise are massive. It's called progressive overload and not massive overload for a reason.

With sandbag training though, you'll still have the benefit of being able to workout practically anywhere. However, unlike bodyweight training, you'll easily be able to add in progressive overload to ensure that you're always improving.

Of course, this won't be because the weight of the bag is always increasing. Usually, the weight of your sandbag will be the same. You can always get a bigger sandbag and fill it with more sand to make it heavier if need be, but don't feel like that's the only way to overload your body with sandbag training because it certainly isn't.

The first thing you must remember is that the resistance will be different every time you train with a sandbag. Even if you're working out with the same 50-pound sandbag for example, that 50-pounds will always feel different to your body even though it's always the same amount of weight technically.

This is because your body will never be able to guess how the weight will move around. Therefore in some ways, it's almost like the overload is built right into the equipment!

Additionally, you can also decrease rest periods, do circuit workouts, add reps, do supersets, etc. to make sure that you're always challenging your body. For example, let's say you're doing an every minute on the minute workout where you're doing 8 front squats with the sandbag every minute.

Don't worry I'll explain in more detail how to do these workouts in a later section! If the workout starts to get too easy, you can modify it to where you do 10 front squats every minute instead of 8. You can also decrease rest periods as well. Using the same workout example, instead of doing 8 front squats every minute, you could do 8 front squats every 45 seconds.

These are just a few examples, but the possibilities are endless. There's no reason for you to get bored or unchallenged with your sandbag workouts!

Reason #5: Great Value for the Price

Another thing that I love about sandbags is that they're such a good value for the price you pay. You can buy a sandbag, or you can make your own.

Either way, it's still really cheap for what you'll get out of it. Compare that to having to pay a gym membership every month or buying equipment for your own home gym.

It can get to be pretty expensive! I know this because I've built my own home gym setup in the past.

Depending on what all you get for your setup, it could easily run you $1,000-$2,000. You need multiple pairs of dumbbells, a bench, a squat rack, barbell, and weight plates.

All of that adds up rather quickly. Compare that to buying a sandbag and some sand, filling it up, and boom you're good to go.

You now have a cheap and durable piece of equipment that'll last you for years and years to come. Having a sandbag is like having your own portable gym with you wherever you go!

Reason #6: Sandbags are Super Versatile

Not only is a sandbag a great value for the price, but they can be used to help you achieve a wide variety of fitness goals. It doesn't matter if you want to burn fat, build muscle, build strength, increase your conditioning, or become more athletic, a sandbag will be able to help you get the job done.

A sandbag will also allow you to work every muscle in your body with multiple different exercises. It'll also be able to work on smaller stabilizer muscles that typically don't get worked with a standard barbell or dumbbell. Don't be fooled into thinking that a simple bag won't be able to thoroughly workout a certain muscle because it most definitely can.

Reason #7: Phenomenal Tool for Conditioning

Lifting weights are great for building strength and muscle, but if you lift for strength, then it's not a good tool for conditioning. This is a trap that I fell into.

I only concerned myself with getting stronger and building muscle. On the outside, I certainly looked like I was in great shape, but I knew that I wasn't.

If I had to run a 100-meter sprint for example, I knew that I'd be gassed. I should've been incorporating more cardio into my workout routine, but I've always hated cardio because of how boring it is!

Not only that but sometimes it can be hard to add strength if you do too much cardio. Luckily with sandbag training, your body will be conditioned for many different activities, and it'll allow you to add strength at the same time.

This is because sandbag training is resisted cardio. When you do regular cardio, there's no resistance to it, so you don't get stronger. On the flip side when you lift weights for strength, there's not much of a cardio or conditioning aspect involved.

However, with sandbag training, you'll be doing multiple different exercises in a short period of time, which will increase your heart rate and increase your conditioning level. You'll also perform these exercises with a unique form of resistance, which will help you to gain strength at the same time. This way you truly get the best of both worlds.

Section 2: 52 Different Sandbag Workouts

Wait Before You Get Started!

If you haven't already, I highly recommend that you visit the link below to download the video demonstration guide of me personally performing every exercise that's in the book. This'll allow you to see how the exercises are to be done, which is way better than having to guess and hope that you're doing things correctly by reading a description or looking at a picture.

https://rohmerfitness.lpages.co/sandbag-exercise-guide/

Here are 52 different sandbag workouts that you can do. Feel free to change the intensity of the workout according to your current fitness level.

For example, if a workout calls for you to do 10 lunges every minute on the minute, and that's too easy for you, then increase the reps to 12 or 14 every minute. You can also decrease rest periods. For example, if you're doing a workout that calls for you to rest 90 seconds in between rounds, then you can decrease that rest time to 60 seconds to make the workout more challenging, or you could even give yourself a 2-minute rest if you need to make it easier.

Also on exercises like lunges, squats, step ups etc., feel free to change the way you hold the bag to make things easier or more challenging. For example, you can hold the bag in the bear hug, clean/front position, overhead, across the back of your shoulders (back position), over one shoulder, or across your forearms with your palms facing up (supinated position).

Any of these variations will work great and feel free to interchange them as you see fit. So for example, if an exercise calls for you to do bear hug squats and you'd rather do them holding the bag in the supinated position, then by all means please do so! Regardless, find ways to adapt the workout to your fitness level so that you're always being challenged to improve!

Side Note: A set is a group of consecutive repetitions. A repetition is one complete motion of an exercise. And the rest period is how long of a break you'll take until you start the next set. For example, let's say you're completing 3 sets of 8 reps and resting 2 minutes in between sets for the barbell squat exercise.

You'll squat down and stand back up, completing the movement of the exercise and one rep. You'll repeat that motion 7 more times for a total of 8 repetitions. That will complete the set and you will begin your rest period. Once your 2-minute rest period is up, you'll start the next set and perform another 8 repetitions.

That will complete set number 2, and you'll rest another 2 minutes. Once that time period is up, you'll complete the final set of 8 repetitions, and then you'll move onto the next exercise.

Every Minute on the Minute Workout

Complete the following workouts by performing the prescribed number of reps at the start of every minute. Then when you complete all of the reps, you get to rest for the remainder of the minute.

For example, let's pretend the workout is 15 minutes long and it calls for you to do 10 squats at the start of every minute. You'd start the workout by completing 10 squats, then you'd rest until the timer reaches 1 minute. Once the timer reaches 1 minute, you'd do another 10 reps of squat.

 You'd repeat this for the duration of the workout (i.e. for 15 minutes in this case). Essentially, if it takes you 30 seconds to complete the prescribed number of reps, then you'd get to rest for 30 seconds. During the next minute, if it takes you 45 seconds to complete the prescribed number of reps, then you'd only get to rest for 15 seconds.

Depending on your fitness level you can vary how you complete the workout. Let's use our earlier example of doing 10 reps of squat every minute on the minute.

If the 60 seconds is up and you've only completed 8 squats instead of 10, you could add the remaining 2 squat reps to the next minute and do 12 instead of 10. This concept is kind of similar to rollover minutes with your phone company except you have to do extra reps!

You certainly don't have to do the workouts in that manner if you don't want to. Instead, you can simply start fresh at the start of the minute.

So if you only complete 8 reps instead of 10 during one minute, you can just aim for 10 at the start of the next round instead of having to try to do 12 to make up for the 2 reps you missed during the previous minute. Then at the end of your workout, tally up the total number of squats you completed and see how you did.

In this example, you'd be doing 10 reps of squats every minute for 15 minutes, which would equal 150 total reps of squat. Let's say when the 15 minutes is up, you only got a total of 107 reps, that's ok. Try to beat this number the next time you complete the workout!

Additionally if you want another way to make the workouts more challenging, you can add in an "active rest" such as holding a plank position for the remainder or part of the remainder of your rest period. So for example if it takes you 20 seconds to complete 10 reps of squat, you could hold a plank position for the remaining 40 seconds that you would normally rest.

Or if you want to make it easier, you could hold the plank for 20 seconds and then get 20 seconds of rest. This is just one example. You could do other things like jumping jacks, squat jumps, push-ups, burpees, or whatever else you like that would be a challenge!

Every Minute on the Minute Workouts

Front Bag Forward Lunges

Workout Duration 10 Minutes

Reps: 5 reps per leg every minute

You can vary this workout by completing bear hug lunges, reverse lunges or put the bag across the back of your shoulders and completing the lunges from there.

To perform this exercise, hold the bag in the desired position. Keep an upright posture with a tall upper body and your shoulders back. From here, move one leg forward until your knee is bent at 90 degrees. Make sure that your knee doesn't extend past your big toe, and make sure that your knee stays in line with your foot. Return your lead foot to the starting position and do the same with the opposite leg.

Sandbag Slams

Workout Duration 12 minutes

Reps: 6 total slams each minute

To perform this exercise, stand with the base of the sandbag at your feet. Most of the length of the sandbag should be in front of your body. From here, squat down and pick up the sandbag, standing up and placing it over one of your shoulders. From here, slam the sandbag on the ground as hard as you can. Then repeat the process bringing the sandbag up to the opposite shoulder.

Sandbag Deadlifts

Workout Duration: 15 minutes

Reps: 8 reps every minute

To perform this exercise, walk up to the sandbag with your feet shoulder width apart to the point where roughly half the lengths of your feet are underneath the sandbag. Depending on where the handles are located on your sandbag, you may need to scoot up closer or slightly farther away from the sandbag. Next, grab the handles on the sandbag and bend your knees to the point where your shins come into contact with the sandbag. This is the key when performing this exercise—you want to make sure that the sandbag is as close to your body when doing the lift. This will put the least amount of strain on your lower back. After your shins come in contact with the bag, keep a straight back (i.e. your back shouldn't be rounded or curved) by keeping your chest up. From here, take a deep breath and pull the bag in order to stand straight up with the weight.

Sandbag Bent Over Rows

Workout Duration: 10 minutes

Reps: 8 reps every minute

To perform this exercise, grab the handles of the sandbag and keep your back straight at an angle of 45 degrees. From here, pull the sandbag up and squeeze your shoulder blades together. When performing this exercise, try to focus more on pulling with your elbows rather than your biceps to target the lats more effectively.

Sandbag Throws (simply pick the bag up and try to heave it as far as you can)

Workout Duration 15 minutes

Reps: 6 throws every minute

This is a great exercise to build explosive power, which is especially great if you're a performance athlete. To perform this exercise, lift the bag up to where it's in front of your shoulders. From here, you'll simply want to try and throw the sandbag as far as you can using both of your arms to throw the bag. Imagine this kind of like how you would make a two-handed chest pass in basketball to a teammate that's on the other end of the court. Obviously, you won't be able to throw a sandbag as far, but the motion is similar except for that the sandbag will be at shoulder height.

Sandbag Shoveling

Workout Duration: 14 minutes

Reps: 5 reps on each side (10 total) every minute

This is one of my favorite sandbag exercises, and it's a great one for building core strength, especially in the obliques. To perform this movement, be in a standing position with your feet shoulder width apart. Grab the handles of the sandbag and swing it from one side of your body to the other. As the sandbag moves from the left side of your body to the right for example, your left foot should pivot to stay in line with the sandbag. The same goes for your right foot when the sandbag is moving from the right side of your body to the left side. It's also important to note that moving the sandbag from one side of your body to the other side counts as one rep.

Russian Twists (one rep equals bringing the bag from one side of your body to the other side. For example, when you bring the bag from your left side to your right side that counts as 1 rep. Then when you bring the bag back to your left side that's another rep.)

Workout Duration 10 minutes

Reps: 6 reps per side every minute

For an added challenge hold a plank position for the remainder of your rest period. This is known as an active rest. You can do this during every minute of the workout or every other minute. Vary it however you like according to your current fitness level.

This is another killer exercise for the obliques. To perform this exercise, sit on the ground with your legs bent at 90 degrees. To make this exercise easier, you can keep your feet on the ground. If you want more of a challenge, you can bring your feet off of the ground. From here simple lift the bag up and move it from one side of your body to the other side.

Push Plank with Lateral Drag (complete 1 up down to complete the push plank, then use the opposite arm to drag the bag under your body to the other side. This will complete 1 total rep. For example, complete the push plank, and then if the bag is on the right side of your body, use your left arm to drag the bag under and across your body to the left side of your body. This will complete 1 total rep of the exercise)

Workout Duration: 12 minutes

Reps: 6 total reps every minute

Here's how to do a push plank: get in a push-up position. From here, move into a plank position to where your elbows are on the ground, and then move back into the push-up position. That's how you'd complete one single motion or rep of this exercise. You simply keep repeating going between the push-up and plank position. After you go from the push-up, to the plank, and back to the push-up position, complete the lateral drag by having the sandbag at one side of your body and dragging it across to the other side.

Grappler Twists

Workout Duration: 10 minute

Reps: 5 reps per side (10 total) every minute

To perform this exercise, grab the sandbag in the bear hug position with the bag slanting across your body. For example the bag should go from your left shoulder to your right side and vice versa when you do this exercise on the other side of your body. From here, twist and crunch your body down towards the side that the bottom of the sandbag is on. For example, if the sandbag is placed at the top of your left shoulder and extending towards your right side, then twist and crunch down towards your right side and vice verse when the bag is on your right shoulder and extending towards your left side.

Sandbag Windshield Wipers (each side you bring your legs to is 1 rep. For example, if you bring your legs from your left side to your right side that's one rep. Bring your legs back from your right side to your left side and that's another rep) and **Leg Raises** (keep the sandbag straight up overhead and complete the prescribed amount of reps)

Workout Duration: 12 minutes

Reps: 6 reps of sandbag windshield wipers and 6 reps of leg raises every minute.

Lay on the ground, holding the sandbag up over your head. Bring your legs to the left (forming an L shape with your body) just short of hitting the ground, then back to being straight up, and then move to legs to the right side, then back to straight, etc. This is similar to how your windshield wipers move on your car.

Sandbag Cleans

Workout Duration: 10 minutes

Reps: 8 reps every minute

This exercise is like a deadlift, except for when you're brining the bag up you'll clean it when you stand up. Be sure to refer to my description on how to do a deadlift for the first part of how to do this exercise. And also if you haven't already, be sure to download the free bonus of the video where I personally perform all of the exercises. You can only benefit so much from descriptions, especially for the more complicated movements such as this one.

Sandbag Clean and Press

Workout Duration: 10 minutes

Reps: 7 reps every minute

This exercise is just like the sandbag clean from above, so be sure to refer to that description and the deadlift description for more details. The addition with this exercise is that once you clean the bag, you'll then press the bag up and over your head.

Sandbag Presses

Workout Duration: 10 minutes

Reps: 10 reps every minute

To perform this exercise, start with the sandbag at shoulder level in front of your body. From here, simply press the sandbag up and above your head. Then control the sandbag back down to the starting position and repeat.

Sandbag Squat and Press (Hold the sandbag in front of your body and squat down, and then once you stand up and complete the squat press the sandbag up. That motion completes 1 rep of the movement.)

Workout Duration: 10 Minutes

Reps: 8 reps every minute

To perform this exercise, hold the sandbag at shoulder level in front of your body. From here, squat down and stand back up. Once you reach the top position of the squat, press the sandbag up and over your head. Then return the sandbag back to the starting position and begin squatting down to start the next rep.

Bear Crawl Pull-Through (perform a bear crawl with the sandbag under your body. When the sandbag reaches your ankles, pull the sandbag through your body to where the sandbag is above your shoulders. That completes one rep. Then bear crawl again until the sandbag reaches your ankles and pull it through again to complete another rep.

Workout Duration: 10 minutes

Reps: 8 pull-throughs each minute

Sandbag Step-Ups

Workout Duration: 12 minutes

Reps: 6 reps per leg (12 total) every minute.

To vary this workout you can complete the step-ups by bear hugging the sandbag, by holding it in the clean position in front of your body, with your palms facing up and the sandbag resting across your forearms, behind the back of your body like in a back squat, or over one shoulder. If you want to hold the sandbag over one shoulder, you can simply alternate to the opposite shoulder every round.

Place a bench or chair in front of your body. Hold the sandbag in the desired position and step up and onto the bench. When both feet are on the bench, return back to the starting position one foot at a time.

Sandbag Side Lunges

Workout Duration: 10 minutes

Reps: 6 reps per side (12 total) every minute

This exercise is the same as the forward lunge expect this time instead of lunging forward you'll lunge out to the side. Refer to the description of how to do a forward lunge for more details on how to do that exercise.

As Many Reps as You Can

The concept behind these workouts is simple. You'll have a predetermined length of time (10 minutes for example) and you'll try to get as many reps in of the exercise(s) as you can.

You'll rest when you need it for as long as you need it. The goal is to increase the number of reps you do the more you do these workouts.

These can also be combined with every minute on the minute workouts to make it even more challenging. For example, the goal may be to try and do as many sandbag lunges as possible in 8 minutes. But then every minute on the minute you have to stop and do 5 pushups. Here are the workouts:

Sandbag deadlifts and sandbag bent over rows

Length of workout: 8 minutes

Perform 4 reps of each exercise and alternate between the exercises. For example, once you complete 4 reps of the first exercise move onto the next exercise and so on and so forth. Try to get as many reps as you can in 8 minutes.

Sandbag Cleans and Sandbag Squat and Press

Length of workout: 8 minutes

Perform 5 reps of each exercise and alternate between the exercises. For example, once you complete 5 reps of the first exercise move onto the next exercise and so on and so forth. Try to get as many reps as you can in 8 minutes.

Sandbag Curls and Bear hug Sandbag Forward Lunges

Length of workout: 10 minutes

Perform 6 reps of each exercise and alternate between the exercises. For example, once you complete 6 reps of the first exercise move onto the next exercise and so on and so forth. Try to get as many reps as you can in 8 minutes.

Note: On the lunges, perform 3 reps per leg for a total of 6 reps.

To perform sandbag curls, simply grab the handles of your sandbag and let it rest at your side. From here, use your biceps to curl the sandbag up towards your chest area. Then slowly control the sandbag on the way back down to the starting position.

Sandbag Shouldering

Length of workout: 10 minutes

Perform as many reps as you can. Alternate between shoulders with every rep.

This exercise is very similar to the sandbag slams; expect instead of slamming the sandbag on the ground, you're simply going to drop it on the ground. Aside from that, the exercise is the same, so refer to the description on how to do sandbag slams for more details on how to do this exercise.

Sandbag Shoulder Get-Ups

Length of workout: 8 minutes

Perform 3 reps on one shoulder before alternating to the other shoulder. Perform as many reps as you can in 8 minutes.

This is probably one of the tougher exercises you can do with a sandbag and it also happens to be one of my favorites. Simply put the sandbag over one of your shoulders and lie on the floor. From here, you're simply going to stand up with the sandbag over your shoulder. You can get up any way you like, but the way I've found to be the most effective and efficient is to fully extend your opposite arm out to where it's perpendicular with your body. Then drive that elbow into the ground and twist your body slightly towards that arm. This should help you to initially get off the ground. From here, stand up, and then gently return back down to the ground. Make sure you complete this exercise with the sandbag on both shoulders. Usually I like to do all of the reps on one side, then switch the bag over to my other shoulder and complete all of the reps on that side. Also make sure that you're doing this exercise on a soft surface to lessen any impact that might occur when you going back down to the ground.

Up and Overs and Bear hug Squats

Length of workout: 10 minutes

Perform 6 reps of each exercise and alternate between the exercises. For example, once you complete 6 reps of the first exercise move onto the next exercise and so on and so forth. Try to get as many reps as you can in 10 minutes.

Note: On the up and overs, pressing the sandbag up from one shoulder and over to the other counts as one rep.

To complete the up and over exercise, start with the sandbag long ways over one of your shoulders. From here, press the sandbag up and over your head to your other shoulder, and then repeat the movement going back and forth from shoulder to shoulder for the desired number of reps.

To perform a squat, start with your feet shoulder-width apart from each other with your feet pointing straight ahead. From here, squat down to at least parallel or lower if your flexibility allows for it and then squat back up to the starting position. Make sure that you don't round your back and try to keep most of your weight on your heels. Imagine trying to push the weight through your heels. Your heels shouldn't come off the ground when doing a squat. If they do, then it means that you're placing too much weight on the ball of your foot and not your heel. Also your knees should follow in line with your feet. If your feet are pointing straight ahead and your knees are following a path at an angle away from your feet, then you'll need to correct it.

Supinated Forward Lunges and Bear Hug Reverse Lunges

Length of workout: 8 minutes

Perform 6 reps of each exercise and alternate between the exercises. For example, once you complete 6 reps of the first exercise move onto the next exercise and so on and so forth. Try to get as many reps as you can in 8 minutes.

Sandbag Presses and Sandbag Bent Over Rows

Length of workout: 10 minutes

Perform 5 reps of each exercise and alternate between the exercises. For example, once you complete 5 reps of the first exercise move onto the next exercise and so on and so forth. Try to get as many reps as you can in 10 minutes.

Push Plank with Lateral Drag

Length of workout: 3 minutes

Perform 1 rep of each exercise and alternate between the exercises. For example, once you complete 1 rep of the first exercise move onto the next exercise and so on and so forth. Try to get as many reps as you can in 3 minutes.

Note: Going down to your forearms and then fully extending your arms completes one rep of the push plank. Once that rep is completed perform one rep of the lateral drag where you'll drag the bag from one side of your body to the other side.

Rotational Deadlifts

Length of workout: 5 minutes

Perform as many reps as you can in 5 minutes.

This exercise is similar to the standard deadlift, with a slight twist to it. Be sure to refer to the deadlift description to know how to complete a regular deadlift. The difference with the rotational deadlift is that you're going to start with the sandbag on one side of your body. From here, you'll deadlift the sandbag up to where it's directly in front of your body. Then lower the sandbag to the ground to the opposite side of your body. After that, deadlift it back up to where it's in front of your body, and then return it back down to the ground on the opposite side. Essentially this is a deadlift where you alternate deadlifting the bag between both sides of your body instead of keeping the sandbag directly in front of your body the entire time.

As Many Reps as You Can Plus Every Minute on the Minute

The following workouts will combine as many reps as you can with every minute on the minute workouts. Refer to previous parts of the book for a more detailed version of how to complete these types of workouts.

As an example, let's say you're trying to get as many reps of the bent over row in as possible in 8 minutes. Then every minute on the minute you'll have to do 3 sandbag squats. These means at the top of every minute, you'll stop the bent over rows if you're currently doing them and perform 3 sandbag squats. Then for the remainder of the minute, you'll try to squeeze in as many reps of the bent over row as you can. Take rest as needed during the workout.

As Many Reps as You Can: Sandbag Shoulders Presses

Every Minute on the Minute: Sandbag Bear Hug Walks for approximately 20 yards.

Workout Length: 10 minutes

As Many Reps as You Can: Russian Twists

Every Minute on the Minute: Sandbag Shouldering 2 reps per side

Workout Length: 10 minutes

As Many Reps as You Can: Sandbag Step Ups (hold the bag however you like)

Every Minute on the Minute: Suitcase Holds 15 seconds

Workout Length: 8 Minutes

Note: Hold the sandbag in one hand for 15 seconds like you would a suitcase. During the next minute, alternate and hold the sandbag in the opposite hand. Alternate between hand each minute. This every minute on the minute workout is different because the length of time it'll take you to complete the exercise is set. Don't let that fool you because it's still very challenging!

As Many Reps as You Can: Bear Hug Squats

Every Minute on the Minute: 180-degree burpees 3 reps

Workout Length: 10 minutes

To perform a regular burpee, you'll squat down, extend your legs out behind you, complete a push-up, tuck your legs back in, squat back up, and jump. With the burpee 180s, you'll start with your body facing perpendicular to the sandbag. Do a burpee in front of the sandbag, except for when you stand up to jump, you'll jump over the sandbag and then turn your body to where you're facing the sandbag on the opposite side that you were just on. From here, you'll complete another rep, and then jump over the sandbag again and then turn 180 degrees to where your body is facing the sandbag.

As Many Reps as You Can: Sandbag Deadlifts

Every Minute on the Minute: Lateral Hops Over Sandbag 6 jumps

Workout Length: 10 minutes

Note: On the sandbag lateral hops, each jump over the sandbag counts as 1 rep.

To perform lateral hops over the sandbag, start with the sandbag facing perpendicular to your body. From here, jump over the bag from side to side. Each jump over the sandbag counts as one rep.

As Many Reps as You Can: Overhead Lunges

Every Minute on the Minute: Sandbag Shoulder Presses 5 reps

Workout Length: 10 minutes

As Many Reps as You Can: Bear Hug Sandbag Jump Squats

Every Minute on the Minute: Russian Twists 2 reps per side

Workout Length: 5 minutes

The jump squat is the same movement as the squat with a slight difference at the end. Be sure to refer to the description of how to do a squat first so you know how to do that movement properly. The difference with the jump squat is that as you're standing back up, you're going to jump off of the ground. Once you land, you're going to squat back down again, and then jump once you reach the top part of the movement. My jumps when doing jump squats with a sandbag aren't maximum effort jumps. Instead I jump roughly six inches in the air or so (just try to get your feet off the ground) and I focus more on rhythm and consistency.

As Many Reps as You Can: Sandbag Burpee Thrust

Every Minute on the Minute: Sandbag Curls 4 reps

Workout Length: 7 minutes

Sandbag Circuit Workouts

To complete a circuit workout, you'll perform all of the listed exercises back-to-back without any rest. Then once you've completed all of the exercises, you'll take the prescribed amount of rest time.

For example, let's say a workout had you doing 10 reps of squat, 10 reps of shoulder press, and 10 lunges with a rest period of 90 seconds in between rounds. You'd do 10 squats and then immediately move onto 10 reps of shoulder press and then immediately move onto 10 reps of lunges. Then once you've finished all of the exercises, you'd rest for 90 seconds and start the next round. Here are the workouts:

Exercises:

- Sandbag Bent Over Rows 8 reps
- Sandbag Deadlifts 8 reps
- Sandbag Curls 8 reps

Number of rounds: 4

Rest period in between rounds: 90 seconds

Exercises:

- Pushup Pull Through 6 reps
- Up and Overs 6 reps
- Bent Over Rows 6 reps
- Sandbag Back Squats 6 reps

Number of rounds: 6

Rest period in between rounds: 2 minutes seconds

Note: On the pushup pull troughs, performing one pushup and then pulling the bag from one side of your body across to the other counts as one rep. And on the up and overs, pushing the weight up from one shoulder up and over to the other shoulder counts as one rep.

Exercises:

- Sandbag Overhead Lunges 10 reps
- Sandbag Shoveling 10 reps
- Sandbag Shoulder Get Ups 10 reps

Number of rounds: 5

Rest period in between rounds: 60 seconds

Note: for the sandbag shoulder get-ups perform 5 reps on one shoulder and then switch over to the other shoulder and perform the remaining 5 reps. And on the sandbag shoveling going from one side of your body to the other counts as one rep.

Exercises:

- Sandbag Pull Throughs 12 reps
- Sandbag Suitcase Holds 30 seconds
- Sandbag Curls 10 reps
- Sandbag Front Squats 10 reps
- Sandbag Rotational Deadlifts 10 reps

Number of rounds: 4

Rest period in between rounds: 2 minutes

Note: On the suitcase holds, hold the sandbag in one hand for 30 seconds during the first round and then alternate between hands during each round. For the pull throughs, each time you pull the bag across to the other side of your body counts as one rep.

Exercises:

- Sandbag Cleans 7 reps
- Sandbag Supinated Side Lunge 8 reps (4 per leg)
- Sandbag Squat and Press 9 reps
- Sandbag Bear Hug Reverse Lunges 10 reps (5 per leg)

Number of rounds: 5

Rest period in between rounds: 2 minutes seconds

Exercises:

- Sandbag Step Ups 10 reps (hold the bag however you like) (5 per side)
- Sandbag High Pulls 6 reps
- Sandbag Rotational Deadlifts 8 reps
- Sandbag Rotational Forward Lunge 8 reps (4 per side)

Number of rounds: 5

Rest period in between rounds: 90 seconds

Exercises:

- Sandbag Shoulder Press 5 reps
- Sandbag Bear Hug Carry 25 yards
- Sandbag Bear Hug Squats 5 reps
- Sandbag Bear Hug Carry 25 yards

Number of rounds: 5

Rest period in between rounds: 2 minutes seconds

To perform the sandbag bear hug carry, simply hold the sandbag in the bear hug position and walk with it for the certain length.

Exercises:

- Sandbag Shouldering 8 reps (4 per shoulder)
- Sandbag Rotational Reverse Lunge 8 reps (4 per leg)
- Push Up Pull Throughs 8 reps
- Sandbag Curls 8 reps

Number of rounds: 3

Rest period in between rounds: 60 seconds

Note: on the push-up pull throughs do one push up and then pull the sandbag from one side of your body across to the other. That counts as one rep.

Exercises:

- Sandbag Shoulder Get Ups 8 reps
- Sandbag Shoveling 12 reps
- Sandbag Deadlifts 12 reps

Number of rounds: 6

Rest period in between rounds: 2 minutes rest

Exercises:

- Russian Twists 12 reps
- Sandbag Dead bug 12 reps
- Sandbag Shoveling 12 reps

Number of rounds: 3

Rest period in between rounds: 60 seconds

Note: Each time you move the sandbag from one side to the other counts as one rep. For the dead bug exercise, each time your leg touches the ground counts as one rep. And finally, for the shoveling exercise, each time you swing the bag from one side to the other counts as one rep.

To perform the sandbag dead bug exercise, start by lying on the floor with the sandbag above your head. Form here, raise your legs up off the floor and have a bend in your knees of 90 degrees. Then slowly lower one of your legs until your heel touches the floor and return that leg back to the starting position. Then complete the same motion on the opposite leg. If you want more of a challenge, you can do the same exercise except instead of bending your legs at a 90 degree angle, you can keep your legs straight out in front of you.

Exercises:

- Burpee Shouldering 6 reps
- Burpee Thrusters 7 reps
- Burpee 180s 8 reps

Number of rounds: 5

Rest period in between rounds: 90 seconds

Exercises:

- Sandbag Hip Bridges 10 reps
- Burpee 180s 8 reps
- Up and Overs 10 reps

Number of rounds: 6

Rest period in between rounds: 90 seconds

To perform the sandbag hip bridge, start by placing the sandbag across your hips and lie on the floor. From here, bend your knees at a 90-degree angle. Then raise your butt off of the ground to the point where your body forms a straight line from your knees to your shoulders. Then slowly lower your butt back down to the ground. This is a great exercise for strengthening the glutes (i.e. your butt) and your hamstrings.

Exercises:

- Sandbag Leg Raises 6 reps
- Sandbag Windshield Wipers 6 reps
- Sandbag Dead bugs 6 reps

Number of rounds: 3

Rest period in between rounds: 2 minutes

Exercises:

- Sandbag Overhead Squat 8 reps
- Sandbag Overhead Forward Lunges 8 reps
- Sandbag Overhead Walk 20 yards

Number of rounds: 5

Rest period in between rounds: 2 minutes seconds

To perform the sandbag overhead walk, get the sandbag in the overhead position and from there simply walk with the sandbag for the prescribed length.

Exercises:

- Sandbag Squat Up and Overs 10 reps
- Sandbag Shouldering 10 reps
- Sandbag Curls 10 reps
- Sandbag Bent Over Rows 10 reps
- Burpee 180s 10 reps

Number of rounds: 3

Rest period in between rounds: 2 minutes

Exercises:

- Sandbag Rotational Deadlift 12 reps
- Sandbag Windshield Wipers 12 reps
- Sandbag Overhead Forward Lunge 12 reps
- Sandbag Cleans 12 reps

Number of rounds: 4

Rest period in between rounds: 90 seconds

Exercises:

- Sandbag High Pulls 7 reps
- Sandbag Bear Hug Squats 8 reps
- Sandbag Leg Raises 9 reps
- Sandbag Shoulder Get Ups 10 reps

Number of rounds: 4

Rest period in between rounds: 90 seconds

Conclusion:

Sandbag training is one of the most overlooked forms of training in existence today. Seriously, it doesn't matter what your goal is, sandbag training can get the job done. It's not expensive and it's a durable piece of equipment you can take just about anywhere and get an effective workout in.

It really is up to you. The sandbag makes it easy for you to train anytime anywhere, you just have to be willing to put in the work. If you do, you'll get the results you're looking for no doubt about it.

If you've never trained with a sandbag before, be patient. It'll take you some time to get used to if all you've ever trained with in the past is dumbbells and barbells. Over time though, you'll get more proficient with the movements, and before you know it, you'll be in the best shape of your life! Don't quit, go out there and be the best that you possibly can!